6 WAYS TO INCREASE FERTILITY IN WOMEN AND MEN.

How to Get Pregnant

MICHELLE C. ROBINSO

All rights reserved. No part of this publication may be reproduced, distributed, or transmitted in any form or by any means, including photocopying, recording, or other electronic or mechanical methods, without the prior written permission of the publisher, except in the case of brief quotations embodied in critical reviews and certain other noncommercial uses permitted by copyright law.

Copyright © (Michelle C. Robinson), (2022).

Contents

Chapter 1:

Introduction

Chapter 2:

Natural Ways to Increase Fertility, Natural Diet to Increase Fertility

Chapter 3:

6 Ways to Increase Fertility in Women And Men

Chapter 4:

Aging Effects in Men And Woman And Trying to Get Pregnant After 35, How Anxiety Affects Fertility

Chapter 5:

Conclusion…… Fertility Tips For Women And Men

Chapter 1

Introduction

Fertility is defined as the ability to conceive a child. Each month they engage in unprotected sexual activity; a couple with no fertility-affecting medical issues has a 10%–20% chance of becoming pregnant; when a woman is over 40, her monthly odds of becoming pregnant drop to under 10%. A woman's age is one of many factors affecting the likelihood of a couple having kids.

Only when many parts are in good working order is conception possible. The conditions for image include the ability of the male partner to produce healthy sperm and the female partner to have healthy eggs. This unblocked fallopian tube allows the sperm's ability to contact the egg, the sperm capacity to fertilize the egg, the power of the conceived egg (embryo) to deposit itself in the uterus of the female, and adequate embryo quality. The embryo's health and the Additional power prerequisites include the woman's uterus and hormones to promote the expansion and development of the source. Infertility could happen if one of these elements is impaired, individually or in combination.

Even though the National Survey of Family Growth, CDC 2002, estimates that 7.3 million women and their partners in the U.S. experience infertility, most persons who try to conceive succeed. That figure represents about 12% of Americans of reproductive age. These people seek help from reproductive endocrinologists. Reproductive endocrinologists are doctors that focus on diagnosing and treating problems with infertility. Should consult a reproductive endocrinologist if a woman under 35 has not become pregnant after trying for a year or if a woman over 35 has not become pregnant within six months of trying.

While a sizeable fraction of the population may have diminished fertility, most people will only need minimal help to become pregnant. According to estimations from the American Society for Reproductive Medicine, 85% to 90% of those persons can regain their fertility solely by medical or surgical treatment. Only 3% of people will require more sophisticated reproductive technologies, including in vitro fertilization, to conceive a child.

The majority of people assume that they can have children. Unfortunately, many people in the United States may experience infertility since the reproductive system is so complex and has such strict requirements for proper operation. Although a sizable portion of people experiences fertility issues, there is more hope for those who experience infertility now than ever before, thanks to growing awareness and developing medical technology.

Chapter 2

Natural Ways to Increase Fertility

How can you go about increasing fertility naturally? What are the natural methods?

The ability to conceive young or be forced to conceive young is the definition of fertility, which is extremely basic and highly complex. That definition implies the power of the female to carry a child to term.

For many women unable to conceive, however, just being able to create would be a joy in and of itself. Until a woman becomes pregnant, she cannot determine whether to carry a child to term.

The reproductive system must function flawlessly, comprising numerous components like the ovaries, uterus, and vagina. It depends on various aspects, including the ability to conceive. Additionally, the endocrine system needs to be functioning correctly. It will be incredibly challenging to get pregnant naturally if your body is not producing the right hormones at the right moment.

For some women, the first step to raising fertility naturally is to examine the functioning of their endocrine and reproductive systems. Others would instead take measures to be in the best possible physical shape to increase their likelihood of getting pregnant and carrying a kid to term.

Most women prefer to start with the natural path to assist conception unless there is some compelling reason not to, such as late maternal age. However, surgical assistance or medicines sometimes help a woman get pregnant.

Eating a healthy diet is a brilliant place to start for you and your partner. We are what we eat, increasing your likelihood of conception by consuming a diet high in antioxidants, minerals, and vitamins. According to statistics, one-third of men and one-third of women are the ones who are infertile, with the remaining two-thirds having some underlying condition that cannot identify.

Fresh fruit and vegetables comprise a large portion of a diet high in all the required nutrients. The first step is to examine your general health and what you consume, as women who are overweight or underweight may have trouble conceiving. Tests to determine the cause of infertility can take months, so it will be in your best interests to be as healthy as you can be during that time.

Being healthy is the most natural way to increase your fertility.

Aiming to Boost Fertility Naturally, you will significantly improve your chances of conceiving and your likelihood of becoming pregnant and having healthy offspring.

Natural Diet to Increase Fertility

These days, a lot of couples are struggling since they haven't been able to have a kid or children. Because of this, many individuals turn to medical treatments and even artificial means. These are not terrible; however, they are pricey. There is, however, a less expensive option. If they adhere to a particular fertility diet, it can boost their chances of getting pregnant.

It has been suggested for a long time that one of the things couples may do to raise their chances of getting pregnant or even to boost the woman's reproductive hormones is to follow a healthy fertility diet.

Dieticians, gynecologists, and other experts' recent discoveries have resulted in a steady modification in the nutritional composition of meals that boost fertility during the past few decades. In the never-ending search for information about the miracle of conception, many mysteries have been revealed.

Furthermore, since particular couples' diets impact their chances of becoming pregnant, pregnancy and diet have long been associated with one another.

One of the many natural strategies to boost fertility has been mentioned: a healthy diet for pregnancy. Additionally, a balanced diet may help to lessen several issues that may result in both male and female infertility.

Endometriosis is one of the issues that a balanced diet for pregnancy reduces. Endometrial tissue growth is a symptom of endometriosis. Abnormally outside the uterus and affects the pelvic region of women.

One of the causes of female infertility is endometriosis. Because ovulation is suppressed during pregnancy, the endometrial implants cannot develop and bleed. Due to the extensive amount of scar tissue and adhesions surrounding the ligaments, fallopian tube, and pelvic organs, it is frequently difficult for the patient to become pregnant. A specific healthy diet for pregnancy that includes vegetables, whole grains, wheat, brown rice, and oatmeal can help to reduce this complication.

Polycystic ovarian syndrome is a different complication that a healthy diet for pregnancy treats.

Women's ovaries can develop cysts due to polycystic ovarian syndrome, or PCOS. As a result, a woman's chances of getting pregnant are impacted since abnormal egg cells are produced.

But this issue can still be treated by adhering to a specific fertility diet plan.

Pregnant women should eat foods high in vitamin A, like squash and green leafy vegetables like lettuce, cabbage, broccoli, and cauliflower. Women should also consider low glycemic carbohydrate diets because they may lessen PCOS symptoms. They might include brown rice, whole grains, and other low-glycemic-index alternatives.

Monounsaturated fats are one of the most advised foods for couples to consume in their healthy pregnancy diet. Given its ability to help couples struggling with infertility, monounsaturated fats are among the types of fat that could regard as healthy fats. Couples should choose monounsaturated fats from various virgin oils, including pure coconut oil, olive oil, and virgin coconut oil.

Protein-rich foods are another advised food that spouses could add to boost women's fertility. But keep in mind that the protein should come from vegetables to prevent other ingredients that could not be necessary for the enhanced likelihood of conception. Beans are among the vegetables that can regard as the best protein providers. They could also include lentils, spinach, green peas, and chickpeas.

Couples should also include low glycemic carbs in their pregnancy diets and the recommended items. As previously mentioned, foods with low glycemic carbohydrate content can normalize PCOS symptoms. Because of this, couples should use alternative low-glycemic carbohydrate foods to improve their chances of getting pregnant.

Last but not least, several studies in Obstetrics & Gynecology indicate that should include goat dairy products in pregnancy diets as they increase the likelihood of fertility.

Chapter 3

6 Ways to Increase Fertility in Women Or Men

It is common knowledge that numerous elements are at play when trying to conceive. I've included six easy actions you and your partner can follow to create a child below. Before reading the instructions, you should be aware that they are based on fundamental research that has been shown to work in assisting conception.

1. The first step is maintaining a healthy weight range, which is of the utmost importance. According to studies, those with average weight are at least 50% more likely to get pregnant than overweight people.

2. Avoid Trans Fat, which is Step Number Two and has much to do with Step One. Stick margarine, fried foods, and hydrogenated oils are all examples of goods that contain trans fat. Naturally, avoiding this fat can help you stay within a healthy weight range, but for some reason, this sort of fat does not appear to agree with your hormones.

3. The third step is to limit your intake of refined carbohydrates and sugar. It aids the body in maintaining optimal glucose levels.

4. Consume as much food high in fiber as you can in step four. Fruit, whole grains, and vegetables are some foods high in fiber. Because it keeps you regular, this has enormous health benefits for the body.

5. The fifth and final step is to exercise regularly. You should exercise daily for at least 30 minutes, and preferably more. Doing this keeps your body in great shape for conception.

6. Sixth and final step: Eat one serving of full-fat dairy each day. Whether it be full-fat yogurt, cheese, or full-cream milk, according to studies, eating these items makes it considerably simpler for women to get pregnant than eating their fat-free counterparts.

So, to sum up, You'll discover that you get that little bump a lot sooner than you anticipated if you keep a healthy weight, eat sensibly, and exercise frequently.

Chapter 4

Aging Effects in Men and Women and Trying to Get Pregnant After 35

The phrase "my biological clock is ticking" is frequent. It shows that a lady is aware of her advancing years and cannot have children eternally. It is best to start a family between 30 and 35 instead of when you are 35.

Nowadays, various factors, such as employment, income, travel, and general business, cause couples to marry later. Unfortunately, even though this seems a sensible choice, it frequently has unfavorable effects. As people age, their fertility declines for both men and women.

The facts are unmistakable, and there is currently no easy fix. Approximately 8–10 years before menopause, women go through a " pause "phase." The fertility of eggs is extremely low during the pause, and the chance of a miscarriage is very high.

Between 1989 and 1993, the Pregnancy and Lifestyle Study, or PALS, was conducted. We could follow the progress of 600 couples trying to conceive thanks to their responses to extensive questionnaires and participation in various lab procedures. We did not become involved in any manner; we observed their actions. It was the first time a thorough study of this kind had been conducted, and the findings were unexpected.

Both men and women had a significant drop in fecundity as they aged. It was shocking at the time because women had previously been held responsible for the entire decline in fertility associated with aging. But we demonstrated that aging increased the likelihood of miscarriage and infertility in both men and women. Coupled with a younger partner, men and women displayed marginally improved fertility.

Everyone has heard fantastic tales of fathers having children in their later years. No one can deny that some of the stories are accurate, but most of these allegations have not been proven. After 50, some women experience normal pregnancies; however, this is the exception, not the rule.

After age 35, fertility starts to fall most dramatically, and the change is highly significant. About 10% of women between 20 and 34 years old are infertile. Between 35 and 39, this doubles to 21%; by 40, it is more than 30%. After age 40, the rate rises sharply, and male aging has a similar effect.

Unfortunately, the rate of miscarriages rises simultaneously with infertility rates as men and women get older. The majority of older couples with problems have similar histories. "We tried unsuccessfully for several months and had given up hope of getting pregnant. We have been let down month after month.

In the PALS trial, the rate of miscarriage was 10% for women between the ages of 25 and 29, 16% for those between the ages of 30 and 34, 23% for those between the ages of 35 and 39, and 70% for those over the age of 40.
It is the typical pattern; these figures are not absolute, and the woman's chronological age does not always correspond to her biological age. In general, the likelihood of a woman who is 40 years old or older having a healthy, problem-free conception is relatively low.

How Anxiety Affects Fertility

Stress is one factor that affects fertility, but many men and women who repeatedly try to conceive and fail are unaware of this. Life has become incredibly complicated, tense, and challenging in this dog-eat-dog world. In addition to the growing expectations for excellence and productivity, the breakneck pace of life in urban centers is hurting people's physical and mental health.

stress and anxiety's effects on ovarian hormones

There is empirical evidence that stressful situations can change a woman's regular menstrual cycle so significantly that she skips a few months of her monthly period. There is still no conclusive explanation regarding the effects of stress on the egg cells that are kept in a woman's ovaries.

However, experts concur that stress hormones can impact the brain's hypothalamus. As a result, the ovaries fail to release the egg at the anticipated time of the month. The egg's implantation within the uterus is problematic in women who are tense and anxious, according to more recent studies.

Stressed-out people have consistently high levels of epinephrine and cortisol, which set off a cascade that affects the release of reproductive hormones in both men and women. Men's sperm counts decline when they are under stress, according to research. The success of sperm production impacts a couple's ability to get pregnant. Men's levels of testosterone secretion are also affected by stress.

The benefits of stress-free surroundings

Infertility experts now advise couples having trouble getting pregnant to make the necessary lifestyle adjustments. The atmosphere needs to be stress-free for the hormonal balance to occur. This proposal is being made in light of successful outcomes from stress-reduction strategies used by fertility clinics. Recent studies support this strategy.

According to one study, stress management approaches boost the development of proteins that help the egg implant on the uterine lining. Another study found that women who lead relaxed lives have increased uterine blood flow, which increases the uterus' ability to promote conception.

Pregnant women are advised to reduce their stress because worry during pregnancy also impacts reproductive hormones. Stressful situations have a link to early births and a higher rate of miscarriages.

Stress' precise function in human conception is still not fully known. According to some research, the effect may vary depending on the individual's susceptibility to stress and is not always present. Others contend that stress related to infertility only increases tension, which in turn causes other issues like anxiety disorders and severe depression.

It cannot deny, however, that many couples who struggle to conceive live in high-stress situations or environments. We cannot conclude that their inability to conceive a child is primarily due to stress. However, we must acknowledge that lowering pressure and anxiety levels has helped couples who had previously failed to thrive.

Chapter 5

CONCLUSION
Fertility Tips For Women And Men

The American Society for Reproductive Medicine claims that 10% of fertile Americans experience infertility. By making lifestyle changes, many couples can overcome the difficulty of trying to conceive.

Male and female infertility affects both. Male infertility affects or is the only factor in the infertility of about 40% of couples. Lifestyle changes can significantly impact fertility. Both men and women will benefit from these suggestions for increasing pregnancy chances.

For ladies

- Use a kit for predicting ovulation. It will inform you of the 24-48 hours before ovulation so you can plan the timing of your IVF cycle. You and your partner should have sex that day and the day after the test is positive.

- Track your body's average temperature. It gives you a record of how your cycle is progressing. By charting your BBT, you can determine the day you ovulate and spot potential issues like low progesterone and luteal phase defects. You can get a free BBT chart in Celsius and Fahrenheit on my website. Monthly Cycle Charts for BBT

- Consume maternity vitamins. It is crucial for the well-being of both you and your unborn child. The likelihood that your kid will have neural tube abnormalities can be reduced by 70% by at least a month before conception, and start taking folate. You can develop a robust placenta that will persist throughout a full-term pregnancy by taking vitamin C daily.

For males

- Reduce or stop consuming caffeine. One or two glasses of coffee maximum each day. If you can, cut out all caffeine. Your fertility may suffer if you drink a whole coffee pot.

- Remain calm and avoid exposing your scrotum to too much heat. Avoid saunas and hot baths, take cool showers, avoid biking, and avoid excessive exercise. Instead, wear boxers.

- Consume vitamins. Take a good daily multivitamin as a minimum. B12, C (500 mg daily), E (400 IUS daily), Arginine, L-Carnitine, Zinc (20 mg daily), Selenium (200 mcg daily), and Coenzyme Q10 are some essential vitamins for sperm health. For men, folic acid is also advised (400 mcg daily). Consult your primary care physician before beginning any vitamin regimen.

- Refrain from sex for brief periods. Abstinence can increase sperm quantity and potency, but abstinence for an extended period can result in an abundance of older, less motile sperm. Stay away from alcohol for no longer than 3 to 6 days.

- Use medication with caution. There is evidence that certain medications can affect fertility. Anabolic steroids, some antibiotics (nitrofurans and macrolides), sulfasalazine (an anti-diarrheal), and ketoconazole are medications to stay away from (anti-fungal).

For the two of you,

- While you are fertile, have sex every other day. The most crucial actions you may take are to have sex at the appropriate time, but some couples forget to do this. The viable period for a woman's egg is just under 24 hours. Some sperm can live up to five days, but most only last two to three. It indicates that your fertile period starts about five days before ovulation and ends a day later.

- Regular exercise. Exercise for at least 20 minutes daily—three to four days per week. Walking is an excellent way to work out if this is your first time. Swimming is a terrific exercise that is simple to get into if you have access to a pool. Men, keep in mind that excessive exercise can raise your body temperature.

- Refrain from using pollutants like alcohol and tobacco and illegal narcotics like cocaine and marijuana. Please do not take drugs unless your family doctor or OB/GYN has cleared them. When a doctor prescribes medication, both men and women should make sure they disclose that they are trying to get pregnant.

- Quit smoking. It needs to be repeated. Smoking can have a severely detrimental impact on your ability to conceive. Smoking harms the well-being of your unborn child and your health. If you smoke, put an end to it right away.

- Eat healthfully. Consume natural, complete foods. Rather than consuming orange juice, consume an orange, for instance. Don't eat anything processed. It entails primarily avoiding the packaged foods inside the grocery store and sticking to the outside aisles where the whole foods are located. Check the label for bread. If it says "enriched," it has undergone processing. Look for whole-grain bread made without processing. Eat steel-cut oats rather than quick oats while eating oats.

- Reach an appropriate weight. While obese men may have imbalanced hormones, with too much estrogen and not enough testosterone, thin men may have a poor sperm count. Obese women have too much estrogen to become pregnant, but skinny women do not have enough estrogen and may not ovulate.

- Ensure that your diet is rich in antioxidants. Tea, fruit snacks like blueberries, cherries, black plums, prunes, and apples, and vegetables like tomatoes, peppers, parsley, and dark green leafy lettuce are some examples of this.

- Sip copious amounts of water. Should consume Half a man's weight in ounces of water daily. He needs to drink 100 ounces of water for every 200 pounds he weighs. A lady has to consume at least 100 ounces of water each day.

- Prevent stress. Even though the two-week waiting period can make it challenging, doing this is crucial for your reproductive health. Take it easy and savor your time together.

- Keep toxins away. Please do not take drugs until your family physician and OB/GYN approve. Avoid using tobacco, alcohol, and recreational substances like cocaine and marijuana.

- Clear of environmental dangers like radiation, lead, pesticides, and heavy metals.

Numerous couples might increase their chances of getting pregnant by implementing these lifestyle change suggestions. While some adjustments take longer to see progress, others do so nearly immediately. Remember that it takes a man three months to develop sperm, so if activities like smoking or exposure to high temperatures have damaged or destroyed his sperm, it may take that long for lifestyle changes to take effect.

www.ingramcontent.com/pod-product-compliance
Lightning Source LLC
Chambersburg PA
CBHW050324220526
45465CB00005B/2117